The Action Guide to How to Stop Worrying and Start Living

A summary and action plan to help you apply the principles
of the classic Dale Carnegie book
How To Stop Worrying and Start Living

The Action Guide to
How to Stop Worrying and Start Living
Sandra Shillington

Table of Contents

Introduction

The purpose of this guide is to help you put into action the following advice from Dale Carnegie in *How to Stop Worrying and Start Living*:

"We learn by doing. So, if you desire to master the principles you are studying in this book, do something about them. Apply these rules at every opportunity. If you don't, you will forget them quickly. Only knowledge that is used sticks in your mind.

As you read this book, remember that you are not merely trying to acquire information. You are attempting to form new habits. Ah yes, you are attempting a new way of life. That will require time and persistence and daily application.

Regard this as a working handbook on conquering worry; and when you are confronted with some trying problem — don't get all stirred up. Don't do the natural thing, the impulsive thing. That is usually wrong. Instead, turn to these pages and review the paragraphs you have underscored. Then try these new ways and watch them achieve magic for you.

Keep a diary — a diary in which you ought to record your triumphs in the application of these principles. Be specific. Give names, dates, results. Keeping such a record will inspire you to greater efforts; and how fascinating these entries will be when you chance upon them some evening, years from now!"

Those were Dale Carnegie's words, and that's why I put this guide together. After reading *How to Stop Worrying and Start Living,* I wanted a summary of the rules in a place that I could easily refer to. I also wanted one place that highlighted each principle with an area to record my application. It's easy to read about concepts like these, but it's an entirely different thing to actually put the ideas into action in your daily life and take a close look at your thought patterns. When I started following along the book using this format, it was enlightening. Here's what I learned about myself: I had always attributed my worrying to being a mother. After all, doesn't that just go with the territory of parenting? Instead, I discovered it started long before becoming a mother. I learned I've always been a worrier. It was a habit I had developed over a lifetime. I was compelled to change my habits. So, I decided to create some daily reminder pages, along with prompts to reflect and record my own journey — which is how this guide came to be.

It is my hope that the following pages will help you also make new discoveries about yourself and apply the principles in your own life. The daily reminder pages include excerpts of the book's key points, but if you don't have a complete copy of Dale Carnegie's book, pick one up. Then use this guide alongside the book to help make these life changing concepts become a habit in your daily life. It's your personal diary to do just what Dale Carnegie said: record your efforts and inspire you to stop worrying and start living!

Today's Reminder:

Live in Day-Tight Compartments

The first thing you should know about worry is this: if want to keep it out of your life, do what Sir William Osier said: "Shut the iron doors on the past and the future. Live in Day-Tight Compartments." What did he mean by that?

A few months before speaking these words at Yale, Sir William Osier had crossed the Atlantic on a great ocean liner where the captain standing on the bridge, could press a button and — presto — there was a clanging of machinery and various parts of the ship were immediately shut off from one another — shut off into watertight compartments.

"Now each one of you," Dr. Osier said to those Yale students, "is a much more marvelous organization than the great liner, and bound on a longer voyage. What I urge is that you so learn to control the machinery as to live with 'day-tight compartments' as the most certain way to ensure safety on the voyage. Get on the bridge, and see that at least the great bulkheads are in working order.

Touch a button and hear, at every level of your life, the iron doors shutting out the Past — the dead yesterdays. Touch another and shut off, with a metal curtain, the Future — the unborn tomorrows. Then you are safe — safe for today. Shut off the past. Let the dead bury its dead...Shut out the yesterdays which have lighted fools the way to dusty death...The load of tomorrow, added to that of yesterday, carried today, makes the strongest falter. Shut off the future as tightly as the past…The future is today…There is no tomorrow. The day of man's salvation is now. Wasted energy, mental distress, nervous worries dog the steps of a man who is anxious about the future…Shut closed the great fore and aft bulkheads, and prepare to cultivate the habit of a life of day-tight compartments."

Did Dr. Osier mean to say that we should not make any effort to prepare for tomorrow? No. Not at all. But he did go on in that address to say that the best possible way to prepare for tomorrow is to concentrate with all your intelligence, all your enthusiasm, on doing today's work superbly today. That is the only possible way you can prepare for the future.

Living in Day-Tight Compartments

Ask yourself these questions:

Do I tend to put off living in the present in order to worry about the future?

Do I sometimes embitter the present by regretting things that happened in the past?

Do I get up in the morning determined to "Seize the day — to get the utmost out of these 24 hours?

Can I get more out of life by "living in day-tight compartments?

When shall I do this? Next week? Tomorrow?

Today's Reminder:

Use the Magic Formula for Solving Worry Situations

Willis H. Carrier, the brilliant engineer who launched the air-conditioning industry, had one of the best techniques for solving worry problems:

"Step 1 - I analyzed the situation fearlessly and honestly and figured out what was the worst that could possibly happen as a result of this failure.

Step 2 - After figuring out what was the worst that could possibly happen, I reconciled myself to accepting it if necessary. I said to myself: This failure will be a blow to my record, and it might possibly mean the loss of my job; but if it does, I can always get another position. Then an extremely important thing happened: I immediately relaxed and felt a sense of peace that I hadn't experienced in days.

Step 3 - From that time on, I calmly devoted my time and energy to trying to improve upon the worst which I had already accepted mentally."

One of the worst things about worrying is that it destroys our ability to concentrate. When we worry, our minds jump around, and we lose all power of decision. However, when we force ourselves to face the worst and accept it mentally, we then eliminate all those vague imaginings and put ourselves in a position in which we are able to concentrate on our problem.

Apply The Magic Formula

If you have a worry situation, apply the magic formula of Willis H. Carrier by doing these three things:

Ask yourself, "What is the worst that could possibly happen?"

Prepare to accept it if you have to. How can you reconcile it?

Calmly proceed to improve on the worst outcome. What can you do to minimize the impact? Your mind is now free to concentrate on the possible options.

Today's Reminder:

Think About What Worry May Do To You

Plato said that "the greatest mistake physicians make is that they attempt to cure the body without attempting to cure the mind; yet the mind and body are one and should not be treated separately!"

Remind yourself of the exorbitant price you can pay for worry in terms of your health.

"Those who do not know how to fight worry die young."

Can you keep the peace of your inner self in the midst of the tumult of a modem city? If you are a normal person, the answer is "yes." "Emphatically yes." Most of us are stronger than we realize. We have inner resources that we have probably never tapped.

As Thoreau said in his immortal book, *Walden*:

"I know of no more encouraging fact than the unquestionable ability of man to elevate his life by a conscious endeavor...If one advances confidently in the direction of his dreams, and endeavors to live the life he has imagined, he will meet with a success unexpected in common hours.

The High Cost of Worry

How can you keep the peace of your inner self in the midst of life's busyness?

Brainstorm some changes you can make to fight the tendency to worry.

List 1

List 2

List 3

Today's Reminder:

Analyze and Solve Worry Problems

Of course the "magic formula" will not automatically solve all worry problems, so we must equip ourselves with the three basic steps of problem analysis: Get the facts. Analyze the facts. Arrive at a decision - and then act on that decision.

If you devote yourself to securing facts in an impartial, objective way, your worries will usually evaporate in the light of knowledge. This can be hard to do when you're worrying. Here's how Dale Carnegie recommends to get the facts about a problem when your emotions are riding high:

• Pretend that you're collecting this information for some other person. This helps you eliminate your emotions.

• Imagine you are a lawyer preparing to argue the other side of the issue. In other words, try to get all the facts against yourself. Then write down both your side of the case and the other side of the case — and you will generally find that the truth lies somewhere in between these two extremes.

From costly experience, Dale Carnegie found that it is much easier to analyze the facts after writing them down. In fact, merely writing the facts and stating our problem clearly goes a long way toward helping us to reach a sensible decision.

Solve the Worry Problem

Get the facts. Analyze the facts. Arrive at a decision

What exactly am I worrying about? Write it out exactly.

What can I do about it? Clarify this by writing it down.

Here's what I'm deciding to do about it:

When am I going to start doing it? Carry it out right away.

Today's Reminder:

Crowd Worry Out of Your Mind

To break the worry habit, here is Rule 1: Keep busy.

The worried person must lose himself in action, lest he wither in despair.

Why does such a simple thing as keeping busy help to drive out anxiety? Because of a law — one of the most fundamental laws ever revealed by psychology. And that law is: that it is utterly impossible for any human mind, no matter how brilliant, to think of more than one thing at any given time.

•BREAK THE WORRY HABIT BEFORE IT BREAKS YOU•
RULE #1 KEEP BUSY

SEIZE THE DAY!

WHAT ACTIVITIES HELP KEEP ME BUSY AND
CROWD WORRY FROM MY MIND?

MY TASKS   MY COMMITMENTS

NOTES TO SELF

Today's Reminder:

Don't Let The Beetles Get You Down

Disraeli said: "Life is too short to be little."

On the slope of Long's Peak in Colorado lies the ruin of a gigantic tree. Naturalists tell us that it stood for some four hundred years. It was a seedling when Columbus landed at San Salvador, and half grown when the Pilgrims settled at Plymouth. During the course of its long life it was struck by lightning fourteen times, and the innumerable avalanches and storms of four centuries thundered past it. It survived them all.

In the end, however, an army of beetles attacked the tree and leveled it to the ground. The insects ate their way through the bark and gradually destroyed the inner strength of the tree by their tiny but incessant attacks. A forest giant which age had not withered, nor lightning blasted, nor storms subdued, fell at last before beetles so small that a man could crush them between his forefinger and his thumb.

Aren't we all like that battling giant of the forest? Don't we manage somehow to survive the rare storms and avalanches and lightning blasts of life, only to let our hearts be eaten out by little beetles of worry— little beetles that could be crushed between a finger and a thumb?

To break the worry habit before it breaks you, here is Rule 2: Let's not allow ourselves to be upset by small things we

·BREAK THE WORRY HABIT BEFORE IT BREAKS YOU·
RULE #2 LIFE IS TOO SHORT TO BE LITTLE

REFLECTION

WHAT SMALL THINGS DO I NEED TO DESPISE
AND FORGET ABOUT?

Today's Reminder:

Observe the Law That Will Outlaw Many of Your Worries

As the years went by, I gradually discovered that ninety nine per cent of the things I worried about never happened. You and I could probably eliminate nine-tenths of our worries right now if we would cease our fretting long enough to discover whether, by the law of averages, there was any real justification for our worries.

"By the law of averages, it won't happen." That phrase has destroyed ninety per cent of my worries; and it has made the past twenty years of my life beautiful and peaceful beyond my highest expectations."

To break the worry habit before it breaks you — here is Rule 3: "Let's examine the record." Let's ask ourselves: "What are the chances, according to the law of averages, that this event I am worrying about will ever occur?"

·BREAK THE WORRY HABIT BEFORE IT BREAKS YOU·
RULE #3 LET'S EXAMINE THE RECORD

THE LAW OF AVERAGES

WHAT ARE THE CHANCES THAT THE EVENT I'M
WORRYING ABOUT WILL EVER OCCUR?

HOW MANY TIMES HAVE THE THINGS YOU'VE
WORRIED ABOUT EVER ACTUALLY HAPPENED?

Today's Reminder:

Cooperate With The Inevitable

As you and I march across the decades of time, we are going to meet a lot of unpleasant situations that are so. They cannot be otherwise. We have our choice. We can either accept them as inevitable and adjust ourselves to them, or we can ruin our fives with rebellion and maybe end up with a nervous breakdown.

Am I advocating that we simply bow down to all the adversities that come our way? Not by a long shot! That is mere fatalism. As long as there is a chance that we can save a situation, let's fight! But when common sense tells us that we are up against something that is so — and cannot be otherwise — then, in the name of our sanity, let's not look before and after and pine for what is not.

No one living has enough emotion and vigor to fight the inevitable and, at the same time, enough left over to create a new life. Choose one or the other. You can either bend with the inevitable sleet-storms of life — or you can resist them and break!

What will happen to you and me if we resist the shocks of life instead of absorbing them? What will happen if we refuse to "bend like the willow" and insist on resisting like the oak? The answer is easy. We will set up a series of inner conflicts. We will be worried, tense, strained, and neurotic.

To break the worry habit before it breaks you, Rule 4 is: Cooperate with the inevitable.

·BREAK THE WORRY HABIT BEFORE IT BREAKS YOU·
RULE #4 COOPERATE WITH THE INEVITABLE

REFLECTION

IS THERE ANYTHING I AM RESISTING THAT IS
INEVITABLE?

IS THERE A CHANCE I CAN SAVE THE SITUATION?

SHOULD I BEND OR RESIST?

Today's Reminder:

Put a Stop-Loss Order on Your Worries

When Benjamin Franklin was seven years old, he made a mistake that he remembered for seventy years. When he was seven, he fell in love with a whistle. He was so excited about it that he went into the toy shop, piled all his money on the counter, and demanded the whistle without even asking its price. "I then came home," he wrote to a friend seventy years later, "and went whistling all over the house, much pleased with my whistle."

But, when his older brothers and sisters found out that he had paid far more for his whistle than he should have paid, they laughed at him; and, as he said, "I cried with vexation." Years later, when Franklin was a world-famous figure, and Ambassador to France, he still remembered that the fact that he had paid too much for his whistle had caused him "more chagrin than the whistle gave him pleasure."

So, to break the worry habit before it breaks you, here is Rule 5: Decide how much anxiety something is really worth.

•BREAK THE WORRY HABIT BEFORE IT BREAKS YOU•
RULE #5 DECIDE HOW MUCH ANXIETY IT'S WORTH

HOW MUCH IS IT WORTH?

HOW MUCH DOES THIS
THING THAT I'M
WORRYING ABOUT
REALLY MATTER TO ME?

AT WHAT POINT SHOULD
I SET A STOP-LOSS
ORDER ON THIS WORRY
AND FORGET IT?

HAVE I ALREADY PAID MORE THAT IT'S WORTH?

Today's Reminder:

Don't Try To Saw Sawdust

Fred Fuller Shedd, had a gift for stating an old truth in a new and picturesque way. He was editor of the Philadelphia Bulletin; and, while addressing a college graduating class, he asked: "How many of you have ever sawed wood? Let's see your hands." Most of them had. Then he inquired: "How many of you have ever sawed sawdust?" No hands went up.

"Of course, you can't saw sawdust!" Mr. Shedd exclaimed. "It's already sawed! And it's the same with the past. When you start worrying about things that are over and done with, you're merely trying to saw sawdust."

So why waste the tears? Of course, we have been guilty of blunders and absurdities! And so what? Who hasn't? Even Napoleon lost one-third of all the important battles he fought. Perhaps our batting average is no worse than Napoleon's. Who knows?

And, anyhow, all the king's horses and all the king's men can't put the past together again.

So let's remember Rule 6: Don't try to saw sawdust. The past is in the past.

·BREAK THE WORRY HABIT BEFORE IT BREAKS YOU·
RULE #6 THE PAST IS IN THE PAST

REFLECTION

AM I TRYING TO SAW SAWDUST?
AM I WORRYING ABOUT THINGS THAT ARE OVER
AND DONE WITH?

Today's Reminder:

Heed the Eight Words That Can Transform Your Life

I now know with a conviction beyond all doubt that the biggest problem you and I have to deal with— in fact, almost the only problem we have to deal with — is choosing the right thoughts. I am deeply convinced that our peace of mind and the joy we get out of living depends not on where we are, or what we have, or who we are, but solely upon our mental attitude. Outward conditions have very little to do with it.

If we can do that, we will be on the highroad to solving all our problems. The great philosopher who ruled the Roman Empire, Marcus Aurelius, summed it up in eight words — eight words that can determine your destiny:

"Our life is what our thoughts make it."

If we want to develop a mental attitude that will bring peace and happiness, here is Rule 1: Think and act cheerfully, and you will feel cheerful.

Let's fight for our happiness by following a daily program of cheerful and constructive thinking. On the next page is such a program. It is entitled "Just for Today" by Sibyl F. Partridge. If you and I follow it, we will eliminate most of our worries and increase immeasurably our portion of what the French call la joie de vivre.

•MENTAL ATTITUDE FOR PEACE & HAPPINESS•
RULE #1 THINK & ACT CHEERFULLY, AND YOU WILL FEEL IT

JUST FOR TODAY

I WILL ...

- be happy.
- try to adjust myself to what is and not try to adjust everything to my own desires.
- take care of my body. I will exercise it, take care of it, nourish it and not abuse or neglect it.
- try to strengthen my mind. I will learn something useful and read something that requires effort, thought and concentration.
- exercise my should in three ways; I will do somebody a good turn and not get found out. I will do at least two things I don't want to do - just for exercise.
- be agreeable. I will look as well as I can, dress as becomingly as possible, act courteously, be liberal with praise, not criticize, or find fault with anything and not try to regulate or improve anyone.
- try to live through this day only and not tackle my whole life problem at once.
- have a program. I will write down what I expect to do every hour. I may not follow it exactly, but I will have it. It will eliminate two pests - hurry and indecision.
- have a quiet half-hour all by myself, and relax. I will think of God, so as to get a little more perspective into my life.
- be unafraid; I will not be afraid to be happy, to enjoy what is beautiful, to love, and to believe that those I love, love me.

Today's Reminder:

Don't Pay The High Cost of Getting Even

When we hate our enemies, we are giving them power over us; power over our sleep, our appetites, our blood-pressure, our health, and our happiness. Our enemies would dance with joy if only they knew how they were worrying us, lacerating us, and getting even with us. Our hate is not hurting them, but our hate is turning our own days and nights into a hellish turmoil. We may not be saintly enough to love our enemies, but, far the sake of our own health and happiness, let's at least forgive them and forget them.

"To be wronged or robbed," said Confucius, "is nothing unless you continue to remember it." One sure way to forgive and forget our enemies is to become absorbed in some cause infinitely bigger than ourselves. Then the insults and the enmities we encounter won't matter because we will be oblivious of everything but our cause.

To cultivate a mental attitude that will bring you peace and happiness, remember that Rule 2 is: Let's never try to get even with our enemies because if we do we will hurt ourselves far more than we hurt them. Let's do as General Eisenhower did: let's never waste a minute thinking about people we don't like.

•MENTAL ATTITUDE FOR PEACE & HAPPINESS•
RULE #2 DON'T TRY TO GET EVEN

LOVE YOURSELF

ARE YOU PERMITTING OTHER PEOPLE'S ACTIONS TO CONTROL YOUR HAPPINESS?

WHAT DO YOU NEED TO
FORGIVE AND FORGET?

IS HATE EXHAUSTING YOU?

WHAT HIGHER CAUSE THAT'S BIGGER THAN YOURSELF CAN
YOU SPEND YOUR TIME ON?

Today's Reminder:

Practice Joyful Giving

Let's remember that the only way to find happiness is not to expect gratitude, but to give for the inner joy of giving.

Ingratitude is natural — like weeds. Gratitude is like a rose. It has to be fed and watered and cultivated and loved and protected. Let's remember that gratitude is a "cultivated" trait; so if we want our children to be grateful, we must train them to be grateful.

Human nature has always been human nature — and it probably won't change in your lifetime. So why not accept it? Why not be as realistic about it as was old Marcus Aurelius, one of the wisest men who ever ruled the Roman Empire. He wrote in his diary one day: "I am going to meet people today who talk too much — people who are selfish, egotistical, ungrateful. But I won't be surprised or disturbed, for I couldn't imagine a world without such people."

It is natural for people to forget to be grateful; so, if we go around expecting gratitude, we are headed straight for a lot of heartaches.

To avoid resentment and worry over ingratitude, here is Rule 3: Instead of worrying about ingratitude, let's expect it. Give for the inner joy it brings.

•MENTAL ATTITUDE FOR PEACE & HAPPINESS•
RULE #3 GIVE FOR THE INNER JOY IT BRINGS

JOYFUL GIVING CHALLENGE

WRITE HOW YOU GIVE IN THESE WAYS EACH WEEK:

SPEND $5 ON SOMEONE YOU
DON'T KNOW

LISTEN TO A FRIEND OR FAMILY
MEMBER

GIVE A PORTION OF YOUR TIME TO HELP SOMEONE ELSE

Today's Reminder:

Would You Take A Million Dollars For What You Have?

"I had the blues because I had no shoes,

Until upon the street, I met a man who had no feet."

About ninety per cent of the things in our lives are right and about ten per cent are wrong. If we want to be happy, all we have to do is to concentrate on the ninety percent that are right and ignore the ten percent that are wrong. If we want to be worried and bitter and have stomach ulcers, all we have to do is to concentrate on the ten percent that are wrong and ignore the ninety percent that are glorious.

If we want to stop worrying and start living, Rule 4 is: Count your blessings — not your troubles!

•MENTAL ATTITUDE FOR PEACE & HAPPINESS•
RULE #4 COUNT YOUR BLESSINGS NOT YOUR TROUBLES

PRACTICE GRATITUDE

LIST 3 THINGS YOU TAKE
FOR GRANTED BUT ARE
ACTUALLY THANKFUL FOR

LIST 3 PEOPLE WHO HAVE
HAD A POSITIVE
INFLUENCE ON YOUR LIFE

WHAT IS THE ONE THING IN YOUR LIFE YOU ARE MOST
GRATEFUL FOR?

Today's Reminder:

Find Yourself and Be Yourself: Remember There Is No One Else on Earth Like You

You are something new in this world. Be glad of it. Make the most of what nature gave you. In the last analysis, all art is autobiographical. You can sing only what you are. You can paint only what you are. You must be what your experiences, your environment, and your heredity have made you.

For better or for worse, you must cultivate your own little garden. For better or for worse, you must play your own little instrument in the orchestra of life.

To cultivate a mental attitude that will bring us peace and freedom from worry, Rule 5 is: Let's not imitate others. Let's find ourselves and be ourselves.

•MENTAL ATTITUDE FOR PEACE & HAPPINESS•
RULE #5 FIND YOURSELF, BE YOURSELF

WHAT MAKES YOU, YOU?

WHAT MAKES YOU FEEL
ENERGIZED OR PROUD?

WHAT QUALITIES DO YOU
LIKE IN YOURSELF?

LIST THE THINGS YOU LOVE TO DO.
WHAT COMMON THEMES DO YOU SEE?

Today's Reminder:

If You Have A Lemon, Make Lemonade

When the wise man is handed a lemon, he says: "What lesson can I learn from this misfortune? How can I improve my situation? How can I turn this lemon into a lemonade?"

The more I have studied the careers of men of achievement the more deeply I have been convinced that a surprisingly large number of them succeeded because they started out with handicaps that spurred them on to great endeavor and great rewards.

Suppose we are so discouraged that we feel there is no hope of our ever being able to turn our lemons into lemonade — then here are two reasons why we ought to try, anyway — two reasons why we have everything to gain and nothing to lose.

Reason One: We may succeed.
Reason Two: Even if we don't succeed, the mere attempt to turn our minus into a plus will cause us to look forward instead of backward; it will replace negative thoughts with positive thoughts; it will release creative energy and spur us to get so busy that we won't have either the time or the inclination to mourn over what is past and for ever gone.

So, to cultivate a mental attitude that will bring us peace and happiness, here is Rule 6:

When fate hands us a lemon, let's try to make lemonade.

•MENTAL ATTITUDE FOR PEACE & HAPPINESS•
RULE #6 WHEN FATE GIVES A LEMON, MAKE LEMONADE

BRAINSTORM

HOW YOU CAN MAKE LEMONADE FROM YOUR LEMON?
WRITE ANYTHING THAT COMES TO MIND.

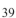

Today's Reminder:

Follow the Prescription for Depression

You can be cured from depression in fourteen days if you follow this prescription: Try to think every day how you can please someone.

Do a good deed every day. And what is a good deed? "A good deed," said the prophet Mohammed, "is one that brings a smile of joy to the face of another."

Why will doing a good deed every day produce such astounding efforts on the doer? Because trying to please others will cause us to stop thinking of ourselves: the very thing that produces worry and fear and depression.

What's in it for you? Much greater happiness! Greater satisfaction, and pride in yourself! Aristotle called this kind of attitude "enlightened selfishness." Zoroaster said, "Doing good to others is not a duty. It is a joy, for it increases your own health and happiness." And Benjamin Franklin summed it up very simply — "When you are good to others," said Franklin, "you are best to yourself."

Let's forget our own unhappiness — by trying to create a little happiness for others. So if you want to banish worry and cultivate peace and happiness, here is Rule 7: Forget yourself by becoming interested in others. Do every day a good deed that will put a smile of joy on someone's face.

•MENTAL ATTITUDE FOR PEACE & HAPPINESS•
RULE #7 BECOME INTERESTED IN OTHERS

START HERE

WHAT GOOD DEED CAN YOU DO THAT WILL PUT A SMILE
ON SOMEONE'S FACE? HERE ARE A FEW IDEAS:

Smile and be friendly.
Volunteer for a charity.
Teach something you know to someone else.
Stop and help someone out.
Do a chore.
Send a thoughtful note.
Tutor a child.
Send a care package.
Visit an elderly person.
Offer to babysit.
Make a meal.
Show appreciation.
Donate food.
Lend an ear.

Today's Reminder:

Try the Perfect Way to Conquer Worry

If we are worried and anxious — why not try prayer? Why not, as Immanuel Kant said, "accept a belief in God because we need such a belief?" Why not link ourselves now "with the inexhaustible motive power that spins the universe?" Even if you are not a religious person by nature or training — even if you are an out-and-out sceptic — prayer can help you much more than you believe, for it is a practical thing. What do I mean, practical? I mean that prayer fulfills these three very basic psychological needs which all people share, whether they believe in God or not:

Prayer helps us to put into words exactly what is troubling us. Prayer gives us a sense of sharing our burdens, of not being alone. Prayer puts into force an active principle of doing. A world famous scientist said: "Prayer is the most powerful form of energy one can generate."

It gives me faith, hope, and courage. It banishes tensions, anxieties, fears, and worries. It gives purpose to my life — and direction. It vastly improves my happiness. It gives me abounding health. It helps me to create for myself "an oasis of peace amidst the whirling sands of life."

So why not make use of it? Call it God or Allah or Spirit — why quarrel with definitions as long as the mysterious powers of nature take us in hand?

Give Prayer a Try

An oasis of peace amidst the whirling sands of life...

God, when my heart is overwhelmed, overwhelm me with Your peace...

Thank you for your voice that breaks through the greatest wind and storm swirling around us, and whispers "Peace, be still."

Give me the ability to trust you more, give me a heart that finds rest in your presence, and give me the wisdom to seek peace and pursue it.

God, I come before you ready to pour out my worries, anxieties and fears at Your feet.

Today's Reminder:

No One Ever Kicks A Dead Dog

What American do you suppose was denounced as a "hypocrite," "an imposter," and as "little better than a murderer? "

A newspaper cartoon depicted him on a guillotine, the big knife ready to cut off his head. Crowds jeered at him and hissed him as he rode through the street. Who was he? George Washington.

When you are criticized, remember that it is often done because it gives the kicker a feeling of importance.

It often means that you are accomplishing something and are worthy of attention.

Many people get a sense of savage satisfaction out of denouncing those who are better educated, or they are or more successful.

If we are tempted to be worried about unjust criticism, here is Rule 1: Remember that unjust criticism is often a disguised compliment. Remember that no one ever kicks a dead dog.

•PREVENT WORRYING ABOUT CRITICISM•
RULE #1 CRITICISM IS OFTEN A DISGUISED COMPLIMENT

DON'T BRING ME DOWN

ARE YOU ACCOMPLISHING SOMETHING WORTHY OF ATTENTION?

I can't keep people
from criticizing me unjustly, but I can do something
infinitely more important:
I can determine whether I will let the
unjust condemnation disturb me.

NOTES TO SELF:

_____
_____
_____
_____
_____
_____
_____
_____

Today's Reminder:

Do This — And Unjust Criticism Can't Hurt You

I discovered years ago that although I couldn't keep people from criticizing me unjustly, I could do something infinitely more important: I could determine whether I would let the unjust condemnation disturb me.

Lincoln might have broken under the strain of the Civil War if he hadn't learned the folly of trying to answer all his savage critics. He finally said: "If I were to try to read, much less to answer, all the attacks made on me, this shop might as well be closed for any other business. I do the very best I know how — the very best I can; and I mean to keep on doing so until the end. If the end brings me out all right, then what is said against me won't matter. If the end brings me out wrong, then ten angels swearing I was right would make no difference."

When you are unjustly criticized, remember Rule 2: Do the very best you can, and then put up your old umbrella and keep the rain of criticism from running down the back of your neck.

·PREVENT WORRYING ABOUT CRITICISM·
RULE #2 DO YOUR BEST & PUT UP YOUR UMBRELLA

DO YOUR BEST

YOUR CRITICS AREN'T THINKING OF YOU.
THEY'RE THINKING ABOUT THEMSELVES.

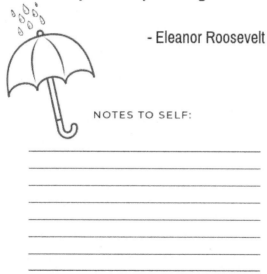

"Never be bothered by what people say,
as long as you know
in your heart you are right."

- Eleanor Roosevelt

NOTES TO SELF:

_____
_____
_____
_____
_____
_____
_____
_____

Today's Reminder:

Be Open to Constructive Criticism

I have a folder in my private filing cabinet marked "FID" — short for "Fool Things I Have Done." I put in that folder written records of the fool things I have been guilty of.

When I get out my "FID" folders and re-read the criticisms I have written of myself, they help me deal with the toughest problem I shall ever face: the management of Dale Carnegie.

I used to blame my troubles on other people; but as I have grown older — and wiser, I hope — I have realized that I myself, in the last analysis, am to blame for almost all my misfortunes.

Instead of waiting for our enemies to criticize us or our work, let's beat them to it. Let's be our own most severe critic. Let's find and remedy all our weaknesses before our enemies get a chance to say a word.

To keep from worrying about criticism, here is Rule 3. Let's keep a record of the fool things we have done and criticize ourselves. Since we can't hope to be perfect, let's ask for unbiased, helpful, constructive criticism.

•PREVENT WORRYING ABOUT CRITICISM•
RULE #3 IDENTIFY CONSTRUCTIVE CRITICSM

FOOL THINGS I'VE DONE

WHAT HELPFUL, CONSTRUCTIVE CRITICISM HAVE
YOU RECEIVED?

HOW CAN YOU BE YOUR OWN CRITIC?

_____
_____
_____
_____
_____
_____
_____
_____
_____
_____
_____
_____
_____
_____

Today's Reminder:

Add One Hour A Day To Your Waking Life

Fatigue often produces worry, or, at least, it makes you susceptible to worry. Any psychiatrist will tell you that fatigue also lowers your resistance to the emotions of fear and worry. So preventing fatigue tends to prevent worry.

So, to prevent fatigue and worry, rest often. Rest before you get tired.

Why is that so important? Because fatigue accumulates with astonishing rapidity.

To prevent fatigue and worry follow Rule 1: Rest before you get tired, and you will add one hour a day to your waking life.

•PREVENT FATIGUE AND WORRY•
RULE #1 REST BEFORE YOU GET TIRED

SLEEP PLAN

HOW DO YOU FIT PROPER REST INTO YOUR
ROUTINE?

My nightly bedtime is:

My wake-up time is:

My relaxing bedtime routine is:

My exercise routine is:

Today's Reminder:

Understand What Makes You Tired and What You Can Do About It

Mental work alone can't make you tired. So far as the brain is concerned, it can work "as well and as swiftly at the end of eight or even twelve hours of effort as at the beginning." The brain is utterly tireless. ... So what makes you tired?

Psychiatrists declare that most of our fatigue derives from our emotional attitudes. We get tired because our emotions produce nervous tensions in the body. Remember that a tense muscle is a working muscle. Ease up. Save energy for important duties."

You can relax in odd moments, almost anywhere you are. Only don't make an effort to relax. Relaxation is the absence of all tension and effort. Think ease and relaxation.

How do you relax? Do you start with your mind, or do you start with your nerves? You don't start with either. You always begin to relax with your muscles. Let's give it a try. To show how it is done, suppose we start with your eyes. Read this paragraph through, and when you've reached the end, lean back, close your eyes, and say to your eyes silently, "Let go. Let go. Stop straining, stop frowning. Let go. Let go." Repeat that over and over very slowly for a minute...

Didn't you notice that after a few seconds the muscles of the eyes began to obey? Didn't you feel as though some hand had wiped away the tension? Well, incredible as it seems, you have sampled in that one minute the whole key and secret to the art of relaxing. You can do the same thing with the jaw, with the muscles of the face, with the neck, with the shoulders, the whole of the body.

Relax in odd moments anywhere you are. Work, as much as possible, in a comfortable position. Remember that tensions on the body produce aching shoulders and nervous fatigue. Check yourself four or five times a day, and say to yourself, "Am I making my work harder than it actually is? Am I using muscles that have nothing to do with the work I am doing?" This will help you form the habit of relaxing. Test yourself again at the end of the day, by asking yourself, "Just how tired am I? If I am tired, it is not because of the mental work I have done but because of the way I have done it."

•PREVENT FATIGUE AND WORRY•
RULE #2 RELAX ANYTIME, ANYWHERE

JUST HOW TIRED AM I?

RELAX ANYWHERE, THROUGHOUT THE DAY

Relaxation starts with the muscles.

Focus on one area of the body - the eyes, the jaw, the muscles of the face, the neck, the shoulders.

Tensions in the body produce tensions in the mind.

Check yourself four or five times a day, and say to yourself, "Am I making my work harder than it actually is?"

Weekly Planner
Pages

WEEKLY PLANNER

Monday

Tuesday

Wednesday

Thursday

Friday

Saturday

Priorities/ Urgent:

Appointments:

Notes:

WEEKLY PLANNER

Monday

Tuesday

Wednesday

Thursday

Friday

Saturday

Priorities/ Urgent:

Appointments:

Notes:

WEEKLY PLANNER

Monday

Tuesday

Wednesday

Thursday

Friday

Saturday

Priorities/ Urgent:

Appointments:

Notes:

WEEKLY PLANNER

Monday

Priorities/ Urgent:

Tuesday

Wednesday

Appointments:

Thursday

Friday

Notes:

Saturday

WEEKLY PLANNER

Monday

Tuesday

Wednesday

Thursday

Friday

Saturday

Priorities/ Urgent:

Appointments:

Notes:

WEEKLY PLANNER

Monday

Priorities/ Urgent:

Tuesday

Wednesday

Appointments:

Thursday

Friday

Notes:

Saturday

WEEKLY PLANNER

Monday

Priorities/ Urgent:

Tuesday

Wednesday

Appointments:

Thursday

Friday

Notes:

Saturday

WEEKLY PLANNER

Monday

Priorities/ Urgent:

Tuesday

Wednesday

Appointments:

Thursday

Friday

Notes:

Saturday

WEEKLY PLANNER

Monday

Priorities/ Urgent:

Tuesday

Wednesday

Appointments:

Thursday

Friday

Notes:

Saturday

WEEKLY PLANNER

Monday

Tuesday

Wednesday

Thursday

Friday

Saturday

Priorities/ Urgent:

Appointments:

Notes:

WEEKLY PLANNER

Monday

Priorities/ Urgent:

Tuesday

Wednesday

Appointments:

Thursday

Friday

Notes:

Saturday

WEEKLY PLANNER

Monday

Priorities/ Urgent:

Tuesday

Wednesday

Appointments:

Thursday

Friday

Notes:

Saturday

WEEKLY PLANNER

Monday

Priorities/ Urgent:

Tuesday

Wednesday

Appointments:

Thursday

Friday

Notes:

Saturday

WEEKLY PLANNER

Monday

Tuesday

Wednesday

Thursday

Friday

Saturday

Priorities/ Urgent:

Appointments:

Notes:

WEEKLY PLANNER

Monday

Tuesday

Wednesday

Thursday

Friday

Saturday

Priorities/ Urgent:

Appointments:

Notes:

WEEKLY PLANNER

Monday

Priorities/ Urgent:

Tuesday

Wednesday

Appointments:

Thursday

Friday

Notes:

Saturday

WEEKLY PLANNER

Monday

Priorities/ Urgent:

Tuesday

Wednesday

Appointments:

Thursday

Friday

Notes:

Saturday

WEEKLY PLANNER

Monday

Priorities/ Urgent:

Tuesday

Wednesday

Appointments:

Thursday

Friday

Notes:

Saturday

WEEKLY PLANNER

Monday

Priorities/ Urgent:

Tuesday

Wednesday

Appointments:

Thursday

Friday

Notes:

Saturday

WEEKLY PLANNER

Monday

Tuesday

Wednesday

Thursday

Friday

Saturday

Priorities/ Urgent:

Appointments:

Notes:

WEEKLY PLANNER

Monday

Priorities/ Urgent:

Tuesday

Wednesday

Appointments:

Thursday

Friday

Notes:

Saturday

WEEKLY PLANNER

Monday

Tuesday

Wednesday

Thursday

Friday

Saturday

Priorities/ Urgent:

Appointments:

Notes:

WEEKLY PLANNER

Monday

Tuesday

Wednesday

Thursday

Friday

Saturday

Priorities/ Urgent:

Appointments:

Notes:

WEEKLY PLANNER

Monday

Tuesday

Wednesday

Thursday

Friday

Saturday

Priorities/ Urgent:

Appointments:

Notes:

WEEKLY PLANNER

Monday

Tuesday

Wednesday

Thursday

Friday

Saturday

Priorities/ Urgent:

Appointments:

Notes:

WEEKLY PLANNER

Monday

Priorities/ Urgent:

Tuesday

Wednesday

Appointments:

Thursday

Friday

Notes:

Saturday

WEEKLY PLANNER

Monday

Tuesday

Wednesday

Thursday

Friday

Saturday

Priorities/ Urgent:

Appointments:

Notes:

WEEKLY PLANNER

Monday

Priorities/ Urgent:

Tuesday

Wednesday

Appointments:

Thursday

Friday

Notes:

Saturday

WEEKLY PLANNER

Monday

Tuesday

Wednesday

Thursday

Friday

Saturday

Priorities/ Urgent:

Appointments:

Notes:

WEEKLY PLANNER

Monday

Tuesday

Wednesday

Thursday

Friday

Saturday

Priorities/ Urgent:

Appointments:

Notes:

WEEKLY PLANNER

Monday

Priorities/ Urgent:

Tuesday

Wednesday

Appointments:

Thursday

Friday

Notes:

Saturday

WEEKLY PLANNER

Monday

Tuesday

Wednesday

Thursday

Friday

Saturday

Priorities/ Urgent:

Appointments:

Notes:

WEEKLY PLANNER

Monday

Priorities/ Urgent:

Tuesday

Wednesday

Appointments:

Thursday

Friday

Notes:

Saturday

WEEKLY PLANNER

Monday

Priorities/ Urgent:

Tuesday

Wednesday

Appointments:

Thursday

Friday

Notes:

Saturday

WEEKLY PLANNER

Monday

Priorities/ Urgent:

Tuesday

Wednesday

Appointments:

Thursday

Friday

Notes:

Saturday

WEEKLY PLANNER

Monday

Priorities/ Urgent:

Tuesday

Wednesday

Appointments:

Thursday

Friday

Notes:

Saturday

WEEKLY PLANNER

Monday

Priorities/ Urgent:

Tuesday

Wednesday

Appointments:

Thursday

Friday

Notes:

Saturday

WEEKLY PLANNER

Monday

Priorities/ Urgent:

Tuesday

Wednesday

Appointments:

Thursday

Friday

Notes:

Saturday

WEEKLY PLANNER

Monday

Tuesday

Wednesday

Thursday

Friday

Saturday

Priorities/ Urgent:

Appointments:

Notes:

WEEKLY PLANNER

Monday

Priorities/ Urgent:

Tuesday

Wednesday

Appointments:

Thursday

Friday

Notes:

Saturday

WEEKLY PLANNER

Monday

Priorities/ Urgent:

Tuesday

Wednesday

Appointments:

Thursday

Friday

Notes:

Saturday

WEEKLY PLANNER

Monday

Priorities/ Urgent:

Tuesday

Wednesday

Appointments:

Thursday

Friday

Notes:

Saturday

WEEKLY PLANNER

Monday

Priorities/ Urgent:

Tuesday

Wednesday

Appointments:

Thursday

Friday

Notes:

Saturday

WEEKLY PLANNER

Monday

Priorities/ Urgent:

Tuesday

Wednesday

Appointments:

Thursday

Friday

Notes:

Saturday

WEEKLY PLANNER

Monday

Priorities/ Urgent:

Tuesday

Wednesday

Appointments:

Thursday

Friday

Notes:

Saturday

WEEKLY PLANNER

Monday

Priorities/ Urgent:

Tuesday

Wednesday

Appointments:

Thursday

Friday

Notes:

Saturday

WEEKLY PLANNER

Monday

Priorities/ Urgent:

Tuesday

Wednesday

Appointments:

Thursday

Friday

Notes:

Saturday

WEEKLY PLANNER

Monday

Priorities/ Urgent:

Tuesday

Wednesday

Appointments:

Thursday

Friday

Notes:

Saturday

WEEKLY PLANNER

Monday

Priorities/ Urgent:

Tuesday

Wednesday

Appointments:

Thursday

Friday

Notes:

Saturday

WEEKLY PLANNER

Monday

Tuesday

Wednesday

Thursday

Friday

Saturday

Priorities/ Urgent:

Appointments:

Notes:

WEEKLY PLANNER

Monday

Tuesday

Wednesday

Thursday

Friday

Saturday

Priorities/ Urgent:

Appointments:

Notes:

WEEKLY PLANNER

Monday

Tuesday

Wednesday

Thursday

Friday

Saturday

Priorities/ Urgent:

Appointments:

Notes:

WEEKLY PLANNER

Monday

Priorities/ Urgent:

Tuesday

Wednesday

Appointments:

Thursday

Friday

Notes:

Saturday

WEEKLY PLANNER

Monday

Priorities/ Urgent:

Tuesday

Wednesday

Appointments:

Thursday

Friday

Notes:

Saturday

Printed in Great Britain
by Amazon